# CLEAN **EATING**
# BASICS

## Your Ultimate Guide to Better Health and Weight Loss

Cindy Hastings

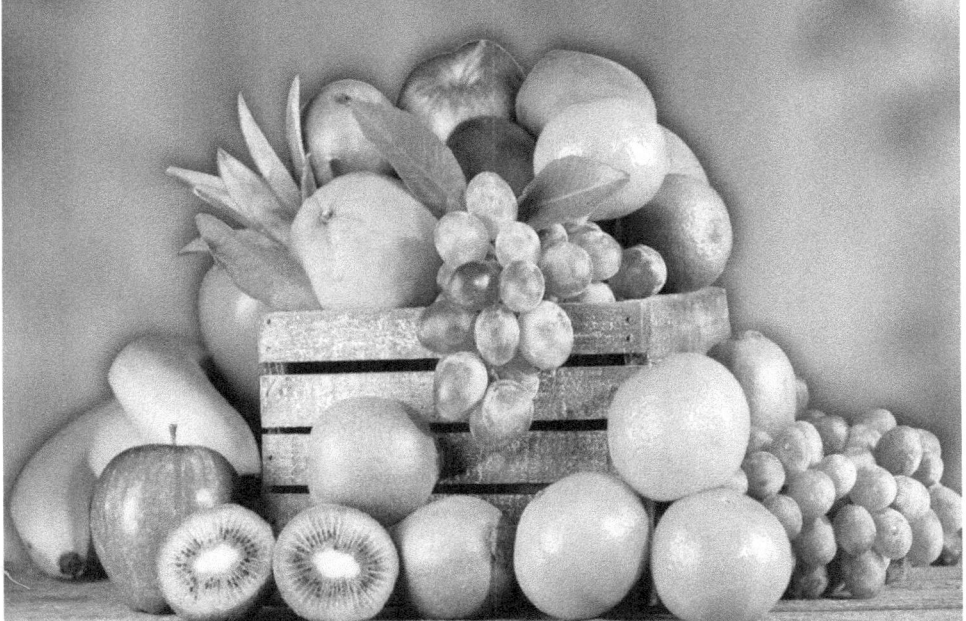

# CLEAN EATING BASICS

## Your Ultimate Guide to Better Health and Weight Loss

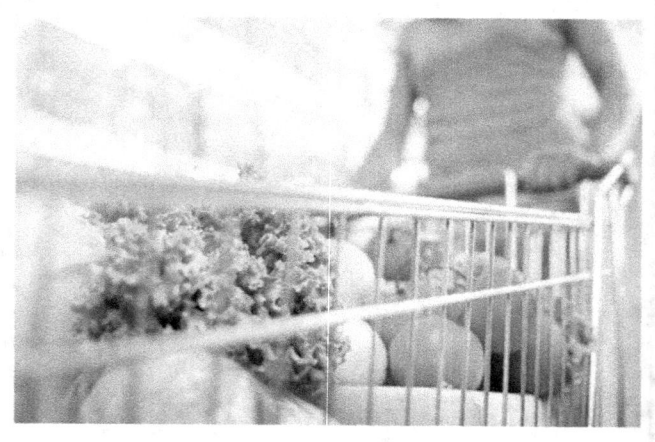

CINDY HASTINGS

# DISCLAIMERS

The book contains information about health and food. The information is not advice, and should not be treated as such.

You must not rely on the information in the book as an alternative to medical advice from an appropriately qualified professional.

If you have any specific questions about any medical matter you should consult an appropriately qualified professional.

If you think you may be suffering from any medical condition you should seek immediate medical attention.

You should never delay seeking medical advice, disregard medical advice, or discontinue medical treatment because of information in the book.

# CLEAN EATING BASICS

# CONTENTS

## CLEAN EATING BASICS

# CHAPTER ONE -

# THE BASICS

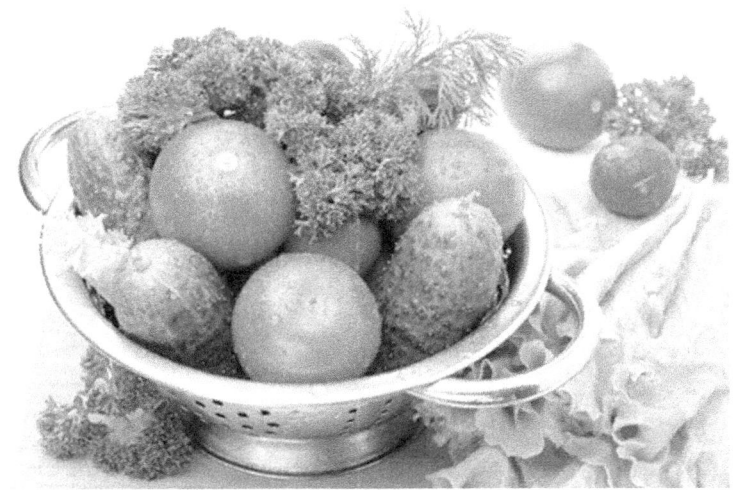

## What is Clean Eating?

If you look around you, you will see lots of people having trouble with obesity. Even though they are in their best years, they are overweight, and their problem with extra pounds is affecting their quality of life. All that refined and artificial food is at the reach of their hands, and they eagerly seek to grab it, neglecting many serious consequences it might have on their bodies. Not only will it hurt their looks, it will also endanger their health and may lead to other health concerns.

First of all, let's clear up something. It doesn't matter if you are in your twenties or your fifties. If you are in the prime of your life, then you should make sure to enjoy your youth to the fullest. In order to do this, it's important that you lead a lifestyle that will make you healthier. You can, like many unscrupulous Americans, choose to eat any old foods you want, because those foods taste so darn good. Or you can put on your thinking cap and start making better food choices, so as to improve your overall health and wellbeing. If you make up your mind about creating a healthy turnaround in your life, your best option is to start leading the Clean Eating lifestyle.

In its core, Clean Eating is an extremely simple concept. It is based on a simple idea – instead of focusing on eating more or less of particular things (such as fewer calories or more protein), your attention is on choosing the food you eat in terms of the road it crosses from its origin to your plate. Food does, indeed, travel a long way to get to our modern day kitchen table. The need for preservatives to keep foods fresh and unspoiled along that journey is part of our modern day problem. The idea is to eat completely 'clean' food, the food choices that are completely unrefined and unprocessed (minimal processing is tolerable) and is as close as possible to the form you will find it in nature. Granted, this might not be so easy to do in the world where modern, processed food is all around us, but with a little effort, you can change your thinking and start to make better food choices. Then, you can start enjoying your food choices in their truest, healthiest form. Now, this is what we call clean eating.

Clean Eating is not a diet; it's a lifestyle. Although there are many great diet plans in accordance with the Clean Eating lifestyle, the main idea is to improve your health and overall well-being. Once you turn your thinking and food choice decisions toward clean eating, you won't be able to imagine living a different lifestyle. You will feel better, stronger, and satisfied with yourself. Most important of all, you will be healthier you than you are today.

Clean eating involves better food choices in each and every food category you can think of. We can begin by saying that each and every food item that you put into your body needs to be re-thought and critically analyzed. Our choices need to be thoughtfully made, and the best choice must be integrated into our lives. Our choices are critical, and here are some categories of food choices where we must begin to make changes if we want to begin seeing some results. Water (bottled plastic, bottled glass, purifier etc.), how we cook our food, all fruits and vegetables must be organic, all meat sources should be graze fed animals, and cooking oils and oil choices must be well thought out as well, cooking pan skillet choices etc.... These are only a few of the critical decisions and changes we must begin to make if we are going to live the clean eating lifestyle. The rewards we can reap in terms of better health for us and our offspring is exactly what the clean eating lifestyle offers. However, do not be discouraged. We must begin to do what we can do. If you start out small, you can begin by making a few changes and then integrating a few more changes down the road. All in all, you must do your best to just start integrating clean eating choices into your diet plan as soon as possible.

# The History of Clean Eating

The History of Clean Eating dates back to the 1960s, when this movement was started as part of a natural healthy food movement. The sixties were the time for various revolutions in culture, and food played an important part in it, as it became a synonym for high morals and values. Later, people developed their wish to have a healthy body and started visiting the gym on a regular basis. Clean Eating has become an important part of people's lives. Numerous dietitians, including Diane Welland and Tosca Reno, spread the word about this healthy lifestyle, and today, it has a huge base of followers, who completely agreed to live this type of life, and it has definitely paid off.

Today, we are beginning to see more and more people paying attention to their health and to their food choices.

CHAPTER TWO-

# TAKING CONTROL OF
# YOUR HEALTH

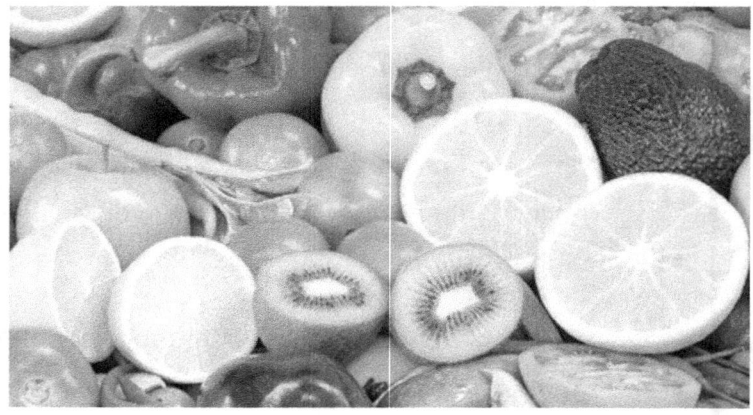

## A Scientific Look at the Benefits of Clean Eating

There are numerous studies about the benefits of various nutrition regimes, and the experts have come to a conclusion that there is no universal nutrition plan that will fit everyone. This is normal, as everyone has different genetics, but when it comes to Clean Eating, there are certain benefits on which all experts agree. First of all, a Clean Eating regime is not forcing any of the food classes out of your diet regime. On the contrary, it encourages a balanced nutrition plan with fruits, vegetables, whole grains, and meat. This way, you can induce enough healthy fats and proteins, while maintaining your main goal, keeping your body healthy.

## The Basic Principles of Clean Eating

If you have decided to try this healthy lifestyle, there are several principles that Clean Eating offers, which need to be respected in order to reap maximum benefits from it.

1. Avoid consuming refined and over-processed foods. This is the foundational principle of Clean Eating lifestyle. The science confirms that modern food is heavily processed, therefore, much less nutritious than the food found in its natural form, whose consuming is promoted by clean eating. This way, you steer clear of trans-fats, which have a negative impact on your health.

2. Turn your attention to fresh fruits and vegetables. Clean Eating lifestyle promotes eating food in its natural form, and fruits and vegetables are a great source of fibers and vitamins.

3. Have 5 or 6 meals each day and make sure you eat something every couple of hours. There are many studies which confirm that eating on a regular basis might encourage better functioning of your body and eliminate the need for having a sugary or another kind of snack, which is often one of the unhealthiest habits people have. You should also make sure never to miss a meal, particularly breakfast.

4. Don't eat sugar. There are numerous snacks and beverages full of sugar, which can cause diabetes and other troubles to your body, and it is best to avoid it. Besides, all those snacks and colas don't have any nutritious value, so cutting them out is definitely a good move.

5. Drink 8 cups (2 liters) of water every day. This is especially important if you're working out, as the body works better, and the muscles grow faster

if they are hydrated. Of course, if you can't drink only water, you can try flavoring it with lemon or making some herbal tea.

These are just some basic principles of clean eating lifestyle. We will discuss them more thoroughly in the chapters to follow.

## The Long-Term Approach to Health with Clean Eating

There are some obvious, short-term effects when it comes to accepting the clean eating way of life, such as feeling more energized and getting better sleep. There are also certain long-term effects that can even go unnoticed. Avoiding sugar decreases risk of type 2 diabetes; not consuming unhealthy fats leads to decreasing the risk of a heart attack and other cardiovascular diseases, and your brain is also well nurtured, so the risk of developing dementia also decreases. On top of all that, antioxidants are highly present in clean food, reducing the risk of cancer.

# CHAPTER THREE -

# STAYING FOCUSED

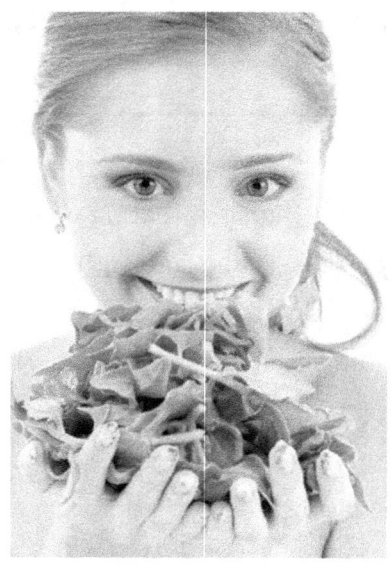

## America a Culture Full of Too Many Food Choices

So many Americans fight extra pounds, regardless of age. Even kids and teenagers develop obesity, which is causing them further complications and affecting their quality of life. The wrong choice of food is definitely to blame here, as the statistics show that obesity has developed, as food with bad ingredients has become more popular. That food is at the reach of our hand, promoted with millions of dollars invested in marketing, and it is draining our energy and polluting our organism.

The fast food industry is the perfect example, as everything that is wrong with American food can be found there, such as loads of fried foods, sauces, and sodas, containing fructose corn syrup, bread, and pies made with wheat, and this is just the beginning. Perhaps you have made a decision to start exercising early in the morning, but stopped by in one of the food chains during the day. By the time you should head to the gym, you won't have enough energy to proceed with your intention. It doesn't have to do with you being lazy; it has to do with food you eat.

And if you think the FDA (Food and Drug Administration) cares about consumers, think again. They seem rather busy with concerns about the health of corporations, instead of worrying about citizens. They are left all by themselves to find an alternative that will enable them a more satisfying and healthier life.

# Join the Clean Eating Revolution It's Growing All Around You

Luckily, people have revealed that all this over-processed food they are eating is impacting their health in a negative way, which is why they have thought of a new lifestyle and started a revolution in nutrition. Actually, it's not a new concept, since it's getting back to the times when food wasn't processed, but consumed in the form the Mother Nature has prepared it for us.

Clean Eating revolution is based on implementing a new lifestyle, where you would consume only clean foods. No, it doesn't mean you have to wash it before eating, but that you should eat it in its natural form, or in a form that is as close as possible to the one that food is found in nature. This is definitely not a diet (although there are nutrition plans you can use for weight loss that are in accordance with clean eating; we will talk about this later), but it's a new way of life. The good news is it doesn't take that much adapting. It means that you should avoid processed foods and visit the perimeters of your grocery store more often, as there you will find fruits, vegetables, and other food that you will consume when living your new, Clean Eating lifestyle. This will, in turn, have numerous positive effects on your health and overall well-being. In the next chapter, we will discuss some of the advantages of this lifestyle.

# CHAPTER FOUR -

# WHERE DO I START?

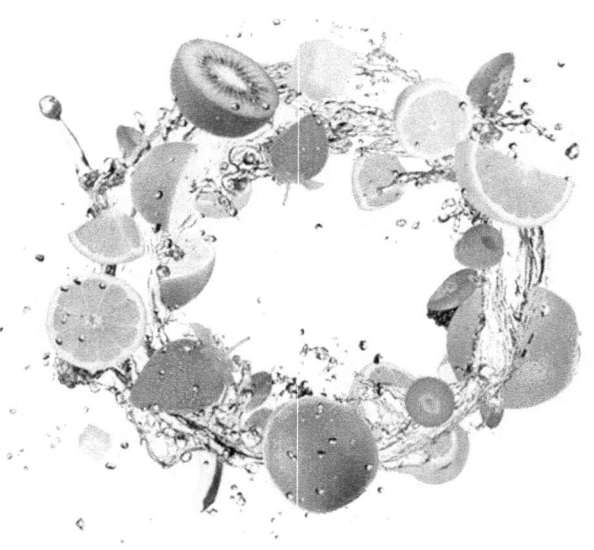

## Advantages of a Clean Eating Lifestyle

When making a change in your nutrition regimen, you are usually motivated by those few extra pounds you gained over the holidays. While this is also a justified reason, there are many more important benefits that Clean Eating lifestyle brings.

You will be healthier – Starting from reducing the risk of a heart attack and other cardiovascular diseases, through increasing your brain function and lowering the possibility of dementia, all the way to having less risk of Type 2 Diabetes, because you have been avoiding sugar, the main advantage of clean eating lifestyle is that you will have positive short-term and long-term health effects. In the long run, the antioxidants in fruits and vegetables you have been taking will fight possible cancer growth. Oh, and ladies, don't forget, your skin will also have more glow.

You will have more energy – Blood sugar spikes, often inducing the fatigue you have been feeling, and that kind of risk doesn't exist when living a Clean Eating lifestyle. Nutrients we can find in fruits and vegetables enable your body to use its fuel more properly, and not only that, a breakfast of whole grains, which are fiber-rich, is exactly what you need to jump-start your day and enable yourself enough energy until lunch.

Better mood – A study has been conducted on two groups of young adults, who have been monitored for three weeks with the task to rate their mood on a daily basis. The group that had been given more fruits and vegetables expressed themselves to be far happier and calmer than the other group. Eating clean is also associated with a better, sounder sleep.

## How to Begin With Clean Eating

They say the hardest thing is to begin. The primary thing you will want to do before starting with the clean eating lifestyle is to discover the reason you are making the change. Perhaps, you have an important life event coming up, and you want to look great, or maybe you're just fed up with those extra pounds and the lack of energy you have, and you feel it is time for a change. Either way, make sure your reasons are good enough to definitely make up your mind, as changing your habits will demand effort.

Next, you should know how much time you are willing to put into forming your new lifestyle. There are studies that claim you can change your habits in a couple of weeks, but you should be aware that any goal worth fulfilling doesn't come easily, and it is the same with a healthy lifestyle. Besides, if you are willing to give yourself to clean eating in the long run, there will be many positive effects on your health.

Next thing is to think about your goals, which should be set in some kind of a measurable unit. It doesn't necessarily mean you need to write down a number of pounds you are going to lose, but you should change statements such as: 'I won't eat so much sugar anymore' with 'I will make a healthy sugarless smoothie every day'. This way, you will have clear goals set and, therefore, better control.

# CHAPTER FIVE-

# DEVELOPING A CLEAN EATING LIFESTYLE

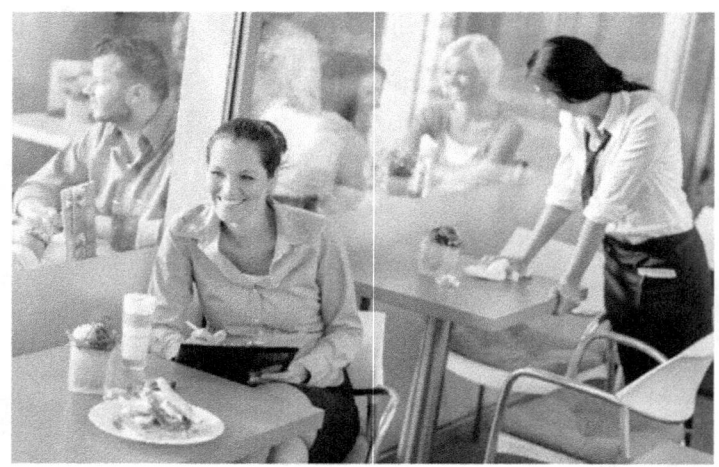

## Develop Your Plan

Great, you have decided to start eating clean. Next thing to do is actually to create a plan for your new lifestyle, in accordance with your life rhythm. Whether you want to lose some pounds or take a turn to healthier life, it is desirable to make a nutrition plan for the period to come. When you are choosing, put in recipes that fit your cooking skills; tasty food doesn't have to be difficult to prepare. Once you get a grip of cooking, you will move on to other meals.

It's your choice if you want to plan it for the next month or just for the next couple of days, but you need to acquire groceries to prepare your meals on time. You can rotate and organize your meals differently for every week, in order to avoid getting bored and full of the same food. Just remember, it's not recommendable to miss a meal, and it is advisable to have five or six meals per day.

## Taking Inventory of Your Eating Habit and Food Choices

It will take a little while to develop a clean eating lifestyle, and down the road, you're going to have to fight urges that your organism has for consuming something sweet and learn how to pass that fast food restaurant that used to be your favorite. It is a good idea to take inventory of your eating habits and food choices, so you can see where there is room for improvement.

## Creating a Clean Eating Grocery List

Once you have planned your nutrition plan for the following clean eating period, you should get to finding all the groceries you need. You will need a grocery list for two reasons — first, this way, you won't forget anything, and second, you will avoid buying processed food much easier.

Once your list is done, head to the local supermarket or a grocery store and head to its perimeters, as this is usually where the real food is. Start by checking out the aisle with fresh products, breads and whole grains and milk and dairy. Move on to meat and seafood, and only then look for other necessities in the center aisle, and choose only what's on your ingredients list.

## Eating Clean While Away From Home

The real challenge of keeping up with your clean eating lifestyle is when you're away from home. The key to pulling this off is preparation. Take the evening before the travel and prepare at least some of your meals for the next couple of days. Yes, it is a lot of work, but it will make things a whole lot easier, tomorrow, when you realize you are too tired to prepare yourself a clean meal or that you even don't have the options for a clean meal at your destination. The most important thing when you are on the road is to plan in advance.

# CHAPTER SIX-

# CLEAN EATING DIET PLAN

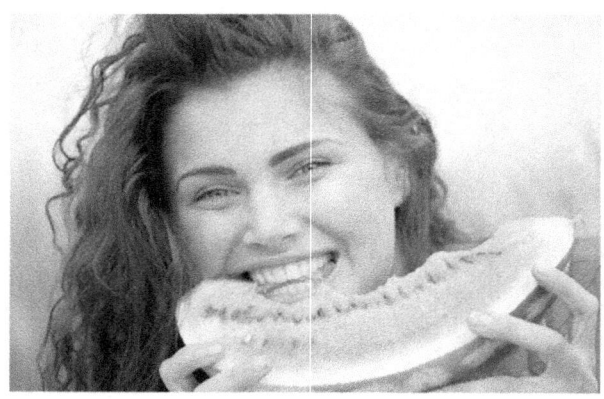

There are so many nutrition experts recommending various diets, which is actually a natural thing, since there is no one-size-fits-all plan when it comes to nutrition. We have already established that clean eating is much more than a diet; it's a healthy lifestyle. However, clean eating is also great if you plan on losing a few pounds. Here's the example of a clean eating diet plan. Feel free to adjust it in accordance with your taste and needs, but make sure you eat on a regular schedule.

You can find some neat recipes towards the end of this book.

# Monday

| Breakfast: | Banana-Coconut Green Smoothie |
|---|---|
| Snack: | Roasted Pepper, Cheddar, and Spinach Egg Muffin |
| Lunch: | Chicken and Avocado Romaine Cups |
| Dinner: | Tuna Melt-Stuffed Tomatoes |
| Night Snack: | Two Dried Turkish Figs with Sharp Cheddar |

# Tuesday

| Breakfast: | Chia Pudding with Pineapple, Mint, And Coconut |
|---|---|
| Snack: | Cup of Blueberries with Unsalted Pistachios |
| Lunch: | White Bean, Cucumber, and Tomato Herb Salad |
| Dinner: | Single-Skillet Chicken Thighs with Asparagus and Red Pepper |
| Night Snack: | Mango Sorbet with Pistachios |

# Wednesday

| | |
|---|---|
| **Breakfast:** | Roasted Pepper, Cheddar, and Spinach Egg Muffins with Blueberries |
| **Snack:** | Chocolate Avocado Pudding |
| **Lunch:** | Roasted Fennel, Asparagus, and Red Onions with Parmesan and Hard-Boiled Eggs |
| **Dinner:** | Baked Eggs in Butternut Squash and Spinach |
| **Night Snack:** | Broiled Grapefruit with Shredded Coconut |

# Thursday

| | |
|---|---|
| **Breakfast:** | Chia Pudding with Blackberries, Coconut, and Pistachios |
| **Snack:** | Cucumber with Ginger Lemon Juice and Hummus |
| **Lunch:** | Salsa Verde Chicken with Cauliflower Rice & Green Beans |
| **Dinner:** | Steamed Salmon with Snap Peas, Garlic, and Quinoa |
| **Night Snack:** | Apple with Unsalted Almond Butter |

# Friday

| Breakfast: | Roasted Pepper, Cheddar Cheese, and Spinach Egg Muffins with Strawberries |
|---|---|
| Snack: | Broiled Grapefruit with Shredded Coconut |
| Lunch: | Niçoise Salad |
| Dinner: | Roast Pork Loin and Butternut Squash with Grapefruit and Arugula Salad |
| Night Snack: | Banana, Chocolate and Coconut Popsicle |

# Saturday

| Breakfast: | AB&J Smoothie |
|---|---|
| Snack: | Peeled Carrot with Humus |
| Lunch: | Roasted Spring Vegetable Salad with Chickpeas |
| Dinner: | Paprika-Roasted Chickpeas with Crispy Kale On Cheesy Portobello Mushroom Caps |
| Night Snack: | Almond Milk Hot Chocolate |

# Sunday

| Breakfast: | Baked Eggs in Garlicky Collard Greens and Sweet Potatoes |
|---|---|
| Snack: | Pear with Unsalted Almond Butter |
| Lunch: | Shaved Pork and Cheddar Sandwich on a Portobello "Bun" |
| Dinner: | Spaghetti Squash with Spinach, Parmesan, and a Fried Egg |
| **Night Snack:** | Coconut and Pistachio-Stuffed Dates |

As we have mentioned, there is no universal diet plan that fits everyone; each and every of them should be tailored to the needs of an individual. You get the basic idea from this suggested diet plan; now, you just need to pick a date when you want to start. Make sure, once you start, you completely devote yourself to a clean eating lifestyle, in order to get the results for which you are aiming. Prepare to put in great effort and don't tolerate any setbacks. You will start noticing the results in a little while and, on top of that, you will feel a lot better than before deciding to live a clean eating lifestyle.

# CHAPTER SEVEN-

# THE BENEFITS OF CLEAN EATING AND WEIGHT LOSS

If you are aiming to lose pounds, you simply must be ready to put some effort and make some sacrifices. For example, you must give up getting out of bed in the middle of the night and visiting your fridge, as well as asking for that extra cup of ice cream. On the other hand, a clean eating lifestyle offers you great benefits – not only you will feel much better with a few pounds shed, but you are guaranteed to enjoy food as much as before, if not more.

First thing you need to say goodbye to are added sugars. All those daily snacks and treats you are used to, such as chocolate cookies (even the ones with raisins) or ice cream, should not have room in your life anymore. Achieving this will reduce the risk for cardiovascular diseases and high blood pressure. If you really have the need for something sweet, go for a natural dessert, such as fruit.

Next thing you are giving up, when going on clean eating lifestyle, is processed grains, which actually means giving up grains that were stripped of important nutrients when refined. With whole grains, you get a higher intake of fibers and other nutrients, which reduces that stomach fat you have been nurturing and has a positive impact on your health, reducing the risk of various diseases. It's simple, actually; you just swap white bread with whole-grain bread, white rice with brown rice, and regular pasta with whole-wheat pasta.

Avoidance of trans-fats and saturated fats is encouraged by clean eating, and these take the credit for a big chunk of those pounds you need to lose. The very idea of following a clean eating lifestyle is enough to keep away from trans-fats, and with saturated fats, you need to be careful about your intake of milk, even if it is low-fat. Also, be careful about cheese. A slice of cheddar cheese here and there is allowed, but try to go with avocado or almond butter, instead.

When eating clean, a weight loss and a healthy nutrition plan go hand in hand. Whether you just want to trim that little fat you have on your stomach, or your bar is set at a higher number of pounds, a clean eating lifestyle is the way to go. You will avoid all those over-processed foods and sugary snacks that lead to having those extra pounds in the first place, so there will be no danger of adding more pounds, especially in the places where you certainly wouldn't want them. Instead, you will consume food that will make you feel better and more energized, since it will not drain your body, and on top of that, you will have a healthy organism.

If your plan is to get fit or you want to boost the weight loss process you are going through, physical activity is more than advisable. Head to the gym to do some workouts on a regular basis, and try to be active during the day, instead of merging with your chair or bed. Find some sports or other activities that relax you, and you will be doing your organism a huge favor. When back from the gym, check out some of the cool recipes in the chapters to follow and enjoy a nice, healthy meal.

# CHAPTER EIGHT-

# CLEAN EATING WEIGHT LOSS RECIPE IDEAS

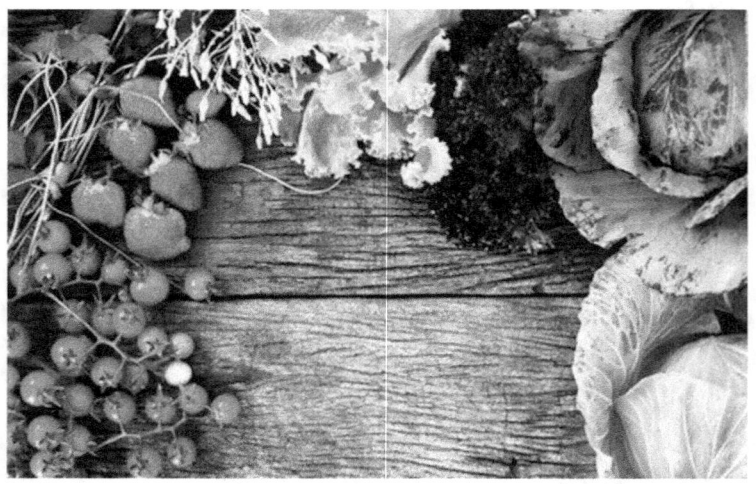

Clean eating lifestyle is, by itself, very grateful, because healthy nutrition is what you need to get rid of those extra pounds you have. Let's take a look at some recommended recipes for a weight loss regime.

# CLEAN EATING BASICS

## White Bean, Cucumber, and Tomato Herb Salad with Ginger-Lemon Juice

Ingredients for 1 serving:  Kosher salt (1/8 teaspoon), olive oil (1 tablespoon), drained and rinsed white beans (about ¾ of a cup), cucumber (one-half), cherry tomatoes (1 cup), parsley leaves (2 tablespoons), mint leaves (2 tablespoons), 1 scallion, freshly ground pepper, ginger-lemon juice

How to prepare: You can make ginger-lemon juice from scratch. Simply cut a two-inch piece of ginger without peeling it and combine it with a zest of 2 lemons and juice of 3 lemons. Put it all in an airtight container and leave it for 10 minutes. You can add jalapeno pepper if you are into spicy food.

You will need a medium mixing bowl for the salad. Put one teaspoon of the juice you have prepared and mix it with kosher salt. Slowly add olive oil and whisk the mixture thoroughly. Add in white beans, sliced cucumber, cherry tomatoes, mint, and scallion.

## Niçoise Salad

Ingredients for 1 serving:  juice of 1 lemon, Dion mustard (1 teaspoon), olive oil (2 teaspoons), mixed greens (2 cups), 1 hard-boiled egg, cherry tomatoes (1 cup, halved), 5 thinly sliced kalamata olives, 5-ounce can of tuna, green beans (preferably steamed)

How to prepare: Choose a large mixing bowl and put in mustard and lemon juice. Whisk it and add olive oil carefully, a drop at a time, while still whisking. Take 2 teaspoons of this dressing and set aside in a small bowl. Add mixed greens to the large bowl that contains the rest of the dressing. Once you have tossed it, transfer to a bowl for serving and put a hard-boiled egg on top, along with tomato pieces, green beans, and sliced olives. Add tuna to the small bowl and then mix everything together. Spoon the tuna on top and season with freshly ground pepper.

**Broccoli and Scallion Frittata**

Ingredients for 1 serving: Broccoli florets (2 cup – 1 large head), low-sodium chicken stock (1/2 cup), big eggs (4-6), 1/8 teaspoon kosher salt, grated parmesan cheese (an ounce), freshly ground pepper, olive oil (1/2 tablespoon), 4 scallions (only whites, sliced thinly)

How to prepare: Turn on your oven to preheat it to 375. Use a small, oven-safe skillet and bring the chicken stock to a simmer. Afterward, add broccoli florets and cook it about five minutes, until broccoli is cooked al dente (make sure to stir from time to time). If there is excess liquid, drain it, and set aside broccoli florets in a small bowl.

Take out a medium bowl and put in eggs, kosher salt, and pepper, whisking it until it starts to bubble a little bit. Add the Parmesan and stir.

Heat the olive oil in the skillet, and when medium heated, add scallion whites. Cook just for about a minute, until the whites soften a bit (don't forget to stir). Add broccoli evenly and then pour in the mixture of eggs. Put the skillet in the oven, which was preheated, and bake for about 10 minutes, until the eggs are nicely cooked and don't jiggle.

# CHAPTER NINE-

# CLEAN EATING RECIPE MEALS

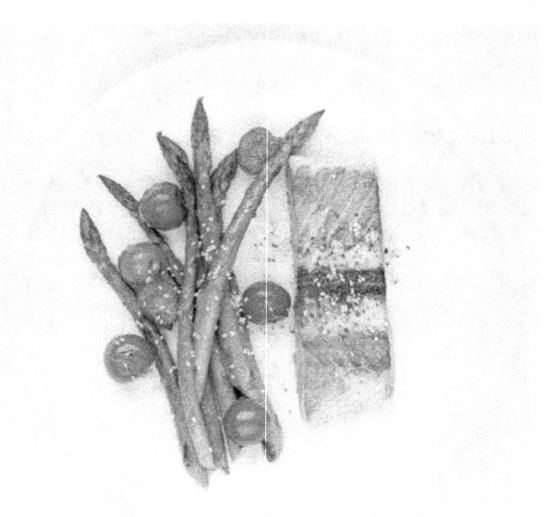

The fact that you are eating clean doesn't mean you cannot enjoy your food. On the contrary, you can enjoy some truly beautiful meals, and some of those recipes are presented in this chapter.

**CLEAN EATING BASICS**

## Collard-Wrapped Turkey Burger

Ingredients for 1 serving: 1 scallion, ground turkey (4-6 ounces), paprika (1 teaspoon), kosher salt (1/8 teaspoon), collard greens (1 bunch, stems removed), canola oil (1 teaspoon), freshly ground pepper, cheddar cheese (1/2 an ounce, sliced), avocado (1/4), beefsteak tomato (1/4, thinly sliced), Dijon mustard (1/2 teaspoon)

Mix ground turkey, scallion whites (finely minced), and greens (thinly sliced), paprika, pepper, and kosher salt in a small mixing bowl. Form a patty, which you will shortly put in a fridge.

Take ¼ cup of water and simmer it in a large skillet over medium heat. Add one collard green leaf and cook it for 20 seconds on each side. Put the cooked leaf on a paper-towel lined plate. Slice remaining collard greens into ribbons and add them to the boiling water. Put the freshly ground pepper and cook for about 10 minutes, until the collards are soft (add water if needed). Transfer cooked greens to a serving plate.

Wipe out the skillet and put it back on the stove. Heat the canola oil and place the turkey patty (medium heat) in the skillet. Cook for about 5 minutes, until the bottom side is browned, then flip and do the same for the other side. When cooked, put cheddar cheese on top and cook until it melts and lay collard leaf on the plate with cooked collard greens, before laying the burger in the center on the leaf. Put avocado and tomato on top and wrap it.

**French Toast**

Ingredients for 1 serving: Egg whites (1/2 cup), unsweetened almond milk (1/2 cup), cinnamon (1 teaspoon), vanilla (1 teaspoon), whole wheat/grain bread (4-6 slices)

Mix milk, egg whites, cinnamon, and vanilla in a bowl and whisk thoroughly. Soak your bread in the mixture, without letting it be too soggy and cook in a non-stick pan over low heat. Before serving, you can mix with blueberries or cherries to get a better taste.

**Spicy Tunisian Grilled Chicken**

Ingredients: Chicken breast (boneless and skinless,1 pound), caraway seeds (2 teaspoons), coriander seeds (2 teaspoons), garlic powder (3/4 teaspoon), crushed red pepper (3/4 teaspoon), kosher salt (1/2 teaspoon)

# CLEAN EATING BASICS

Use spice grinder (or mortar and pestle) to grind caraway and corianders seeds and crushed red pepper. Mix it with salt and garlic powder in a small bowl. Use the rub to coat each side of the chicken 30 minutes before broiling. Use a broiler pan with foil and coat with cooking spray. When you place the chicken on the foil, watch closely and turn it at least once. It should be broiled for about 10-15 minutes.

## Green Gazpacho

Ingredients: baby spinach (100 grams), 1 cucumber (chopped, deseeded), green chili (1/2, deseeded), parsley, basil and mint (1/2 of each), 1 avocado (peeled), 4 spring onions, natural yogurt (200 grams), sherry vinegar (2 tablespoons)

Mix all ingredients in a food processor (you can add a pinch of kosher salt and freshly ground pepper for taste). Add enough water to get a soupy consistency. Add vinegar if necessary. It is advisable to let it chill for at least a couple of hours.

# CHAPTER TEN-

# CLEAN EATING SMOOTHIE RECIPES

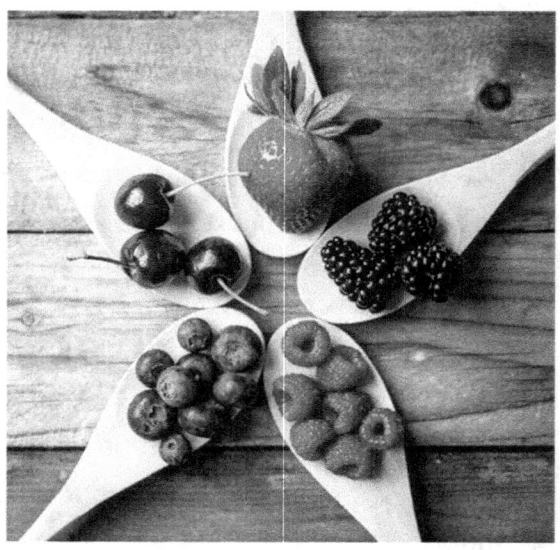

People love smoothies. The feeling when you take a sip of a smoothie, whether it is cold or not, is amazing. The great news is that the clean eating lifestyle allows you to drink them. Of course, you will make them in accordance with the principles of clean eating, which means there will be no sugar added, but with the recipes offered in this chapter, the smoothies you drink will be breathtaking.

**Banana & Coconut Green Smoothie**

Ingredients for 1 serving:  One-half of a large banana, 2 cups of baby spinach, 2 tablespoons of unsalted almond butter, 1 cup coconut water, one-quarter of a teaspoon of vanilla extract

How to prepare: The evening before, peel and freeze half of a large banana. Cut it into approximately 1-inch pieces and then add other ingredients into the blender. Let the blender do its job until the mixture becomes smooth.

**Strawberry Banana Smoothie**

Ingredients for 1 serving: One-half of a large banana, 4 strawberries, 1 cup of almond milk, 2 tablespoons of unsalted almond butter, one-half of a teaspoon of a vanilla extract

How to prepare: The evening before, peel and freeze half of a large banana. Cut it into approximately 1-inch pieces and add it to the blender. Cut the strawberries roughly and then add them and other ingredients into the blender. Let the blender do its job until the mixture becomes smooth.

### Coconut, Pineapple & Avocado Smoothie

Ingredients for 1 serving: 1 cup coconut water, 1 cup pineapple chunks, one-quarter of a peeled avocado, one-half of a bunch of kale, ribs and stems removed, 1 tablespoon of shredded coconut, 2 tablespoons of unsalted almond butter, one-half of a teaspoon of a vanilla extract

How to prepare: The evening before, peel and freeze the avocado. Then combine it with kale leaves roughly chopped into 2-inch chunks, coconut water, almond butter, and vanilla extract. Let the blender do its job until the mixture becomes smooth. Pour it into a glass and decorate it with shredded coconut around the top.

### AB & J Smoothie

Ingredients for 1 serving: 4 large strawberries, 2 cups of almond milk, 1 pitted Medjool date, 2 tablespoons of unsalted almond butter, one-half of a teaspoon of a vanilla extract

How to prepare: Roughly chop four strawberries (if they are tiny, you can add more) and put them into a blender. Add all the other ingredients and let the blender do its job, until the mixture becomes smooth.

## Strawberry, Kale & Avocado Smoothie

Ingredients for 1 serving: 6 big strawberries, one-quarter of an avocado, one-half of a kale bunch, removed stems, 1 cup coconut water, 1 tablespoon of unsalted almond butter, one-half of a teaspoon of a vanilla extract

How to prepare: On the evening before, peel the avocado and freeze it. When frozen, add into the blender. Cut six strawberries (if tiny, add more of them), a kale bunch, and other ingredients and let the blender do its job, until the mixture becomes smooth.

# CHAPTER ELEVEN-

# CLEAN EATING SALAD RECIPES

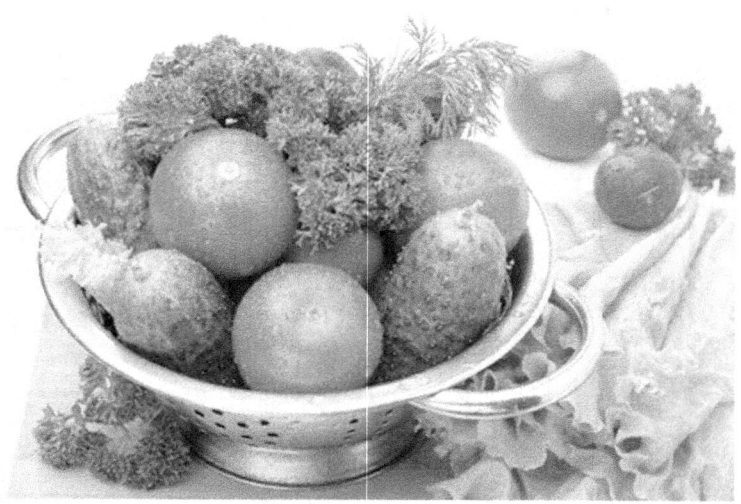

Clean eating is a lifestyle, but as we already established, it can give some great results if your goal is to lose some weight. A great way of having a nice meal, while respecting clean eating and your diet plan completely, is to prepare a nice salad. Here are some recipes you might want to try.

**Egg and Tomato Salad**

Ingredients for 1 serving: 2 hard-boiled eggs, 2 tomatoes, balsamic vinegar (up to 1 tablespoon), kosher salt (up to 1 tablespoon), fresh basil to taste (chopped)

Chop the eggs and tomatoes, as well as fresh basil. Take a medium-size bowl, add all ingredients, and stir them.

**Strawberry Spinach Salad**

Ingredients for 1 serving: Strawberries, spinach, walnuts, avocado, strawberry vinaigrette dressing

Ingredients for dressing: fresh strawberries (1/2 pound, honey (up to 2 tablespoons), olive oil (2 tablespoons), apple cider vinegar (2 tablespoons) kosher salt (1/4 teaspoon), ground black pepper (1/4 teaspoon)

The first thing you will want to do is make the dressing. You do this simply by adding all your ingredients in a blender and mixing them until they are smooth. Once you have prepared the dressing, lay out all your salad ingredients in a medium-size bowl. If you don't like avocado, you don't have to use it. Simply leave it out of your salad. Once the ingredients are layered, add the dressing and mix it all up.

## Cilantro Quinoa Salad

Ingredients for 1 serving: quinoa (cooked, cooled or cold, 2 cups), pinto beans (cooked, cooled or cold, 1 cup), fresh cilantro (up to 1/2 a cup, chopped), juice of 1 lime, garlic powder (1 tablespoon), black pepper (1/2 teaspoon), kosher salt (1/4 teaspoon)

Take a medium-size bowl, put in all ingredients and mix them up. It is advised to be served cold.

## Lemon Almond Chicken Salad

Ingredients for 2 servings: homemade chicken (well-shredded), 1 carrot (grated), almonds (1/4 cup, chopped or slivered), garlic powder (1 teaspoon), coriander (1 teaspoon), ground cumin (1 teaspoon), juice of 1 lemon

Choose a large mixing bowl and put in all ingredients. Stir it until all ingredients are nicely combined.

# CLEAN EATING BASICS

## Chicken and Cucumber Toss

Ingredients for 2 servings: homemade chicken (well-shredded), cucumber (chopped), tomato (chopped), fresh Italian parsley, Italian dressing

Ingredients for dressing: apple cider vinegar (1 cup), extra virgin olive oil (1 cup), garlic powder (1 tablespoon), onion powder (1 tablespoon), Italian herb (1 tablespoon), Dijon mustard (1 teaspoon, no sugar added), dried basil (1 teaspoon), ground black pepper (1/2 teaspoon), sea salt (1/4 teaspoon), honey (up to 1 tablespoon, optional)

Make the dressing by putting all ingredients in a blender and mixing them until they are well-combined. Put the dressing in a storage container, and you can use it for the next 2 months. However, before using it the first time, let it sit for 24 hours. This way, the herbs will have time to infuse into the oil. Don't forget to shake the container before every use.

When preparing the salad, you are left to choose the amount of each ingredient you want as per your taste. Put all ingredients in a medium mixing bowl, put on the dressing and mix them up before serving.

# CHAPTER TWELVE-

# CLEAN EATING SOUP RECIPES

We all love a good soup, and the fact that you have started a clean eating lifestyle shouldn't stop you from enjoying them. Actually, it's completely opposite; this regime encourages soup and offers numerous recipes you can enjoy. Here are some of them.

**Thai Inspired Tomato Soup**

Ingredients for 4 servings: cherry or grape tomatoes (2 cups), fresh lemon juice (2 tablespoons), extra-virgin coconut oil (2 tablespoons), fresh lime juice (1 tablespoon), minced fresh ginger (2 teaspoons), minced clove garlic, sea salt (1 teaspoon), fresh basil leaves (1 teaspoon, thinly sliced), boiled water (2 cups, separately prepared)

Put the tomatoes, 1 cup of water, lemon juice, lime juice, oil, ginger, salt, and garlic into a blender and mix the ingredients until they are well-combined. Add an additional cup of water and blend again until the ingredients are combined. Top it with basil and heat further, if needed, before dividing into servings.

**Chicken Fajita Soup**

Ingredients for 4 servings: chicken breasts (4 big breast cut into small cubes), organic corn (frozen, 1 lb), chicken broth (8 cups, no sugar added, low sodium), 2 red bell peppers, 1 orange bell pepper, 1 yellow bell pepper (each of them chopped), 2 red onions (chopped), cumin (2 tablespoons), olive oil (1 tablespoon), chili powder (2 tablespoons), onion powder (2 tablespoons), garlic powder (1 tablespoon), dried cilantro (1 tablespoon), fresh cilantro (1 small bunch)

Use a large soup pot to sauté the onions and bell peppers in the olive oil. Afterward, add the chicken and cook it, stirring it often. Cook until chicken is almost cooked through, which should take about 5-10 minutes, and then stir in corn. Next, pour in broth and add all the spices. Finally, bring to a light boil and cook it, until you are sure the chicken is cooked through, which should take about 10-20 minutes.

**Cabbage Soup**

Ingredients for 4 servings: 2 sweet onions (diced), 2 garlic cloves (minced), 2 large green bell peppers (chopped), cabbage (1/2 head, chopped), red cabbage (1/2 head, chopped), 4 carrots (peeled, chopped), 2 sweet potatoes (peeled, cubed), 3 turnips (peeled, cubed), vegetable broth (2 cups), water (1/2 cup), fresh lemon juice (1 tablespoon), fire roasted diced tomatoes (1 can), diced tomatoes (1 can), black beans (1 can), chili powder (2 tablespoons), cumin (2 teaspoons), garlic pepper (1/2 teaspoon), cayenne pepper (1/2 teaspoon), cinnamon (1/2 teaspoon), aged cheddar cheese (optional topping)

The first thing you want to do is get a large pot and add chopped peppers, diced onions, and minced garlic into it. Spray it with coconut oil cooking spray and cook for about 5-7 minutes on medium heat. Next, add chopped cabbage and red cabbage and cook it for an additional 5 minutes, while stirring it often. The third step is to add carrots and sweet potatoes and cook for another 3 minutes, and then move on to adding vegetable broth,

# CLEAN EATING BASICS

turnips, black beans, tomatoes, and all seasonings, before cooking it for an additional 5 more minutes. Turn the burner to low heat and leave it for about 20-30 minutes, until the flavor has blended and all vegetables are cooked the way you like them.

# CHAPTER THIRTEEN

# CLEAN EATING HEALTHY SNACK RECIPES

Remember when you were a slave to all those sugary snacks that were destroying your health? Luckily, with a clean eating lifestyle, you gave them all up. However, this doesn't mean you can't enjoy a nice snack. In fact, here are some propositions on healthy snacks you should consider.

**Egg and Turkey Cups**

Ingredients for 12 muffins: fresh turkey breast (12 1-oz slices), low-fat old cheddar cheese (1/2 cup, divided), green onion (1/4 cup, finely chopped), 12 eggs, fresh ground pepper

Preheat your oven to 400°F. Take parchment paper and cut it into 12, four-inch squares. Put one piece in each of the 12 muffin cups. Put a slice of turkey breast over each parchment and use your fingers to line cups with turkey. Take onion and cheese and divide it equally between cups before breaking an egg into every one of them. Sprinkle equally with pepper. Put it on the middle rack of your oven and bake it for around 20 minutes, until the yolk is firm as per your preference.

**Avocado Lime Frozen Yogurt**

Ingredients for 16 servings: 4 avocados (medium ripe), almond yogurt (1 cup), almond milk (1/2 cup, unsweetened), honey (1/2 cup), lime juice (1/2 cup), sea salt

Cut avocados in half, remove pits, and scoop the flesh out from skins using a spoon. You will need to fill 3 cups with cut chunks of flesh (they should be big chunks). Put all ingredients fruit into a food processor and process them until they are well combined. Make sure to stop mixer every 30 seconds in order to scrape down the sides of the bowl. Put the mixture in a container, which can be frozen, and put it in the freezer for 2-3 hours. You can take it out after 30 minutes to scrape the edges with a spatula and mix it with a whisk. Once it is frozen, take it out and serve yogurt scoops, optionally adding tropical fruit chunks before serving.

# CLEAN EATING BASICS

## Sweet and Crunchy Guacamole

Ingredients for 10 servings: unsalted cashews (1/4 cup, raw), 2 avocados (halved, peeled and pitted), Greek yogurt (6 oz, nonfat, plain), fresh lime juice (2 tablespoons), fresh cilantro (1/4 cup, chopped), sea salt (1/2 teaspoon), cranberries (2 tablespoons, unsweetened), mango (1/2 cup, peeled, pitted and finely diced), jicama (1/2 cup, peeled and finely chopped), unsalted pepitas (2 tablespoons, dry-roasted)

Heat a small skillet over medium heat. Put in cashews and toast for approximately 7 minutes. Make sure to shake the pan, occasionally, and when they become lightly browned, remove the cashews from the heat. Take a big bowl, put in avocados and yogurt, and mash them with a fork until they become almost smooth. Put in lime juice, salt, and cilantro and stir. Move cashews to a cutting board, add cranberries and chop them roughly. Once chopped, put it in the avocado mixture and stir. Add mango, pepitas, and jicama and stir again until the ingredients are well-combined. Put it in the refrigerator to cool and use it within three days.

# CHAPTER FOURTEEN-

# CLEAN EATING DESSERT RECIPES

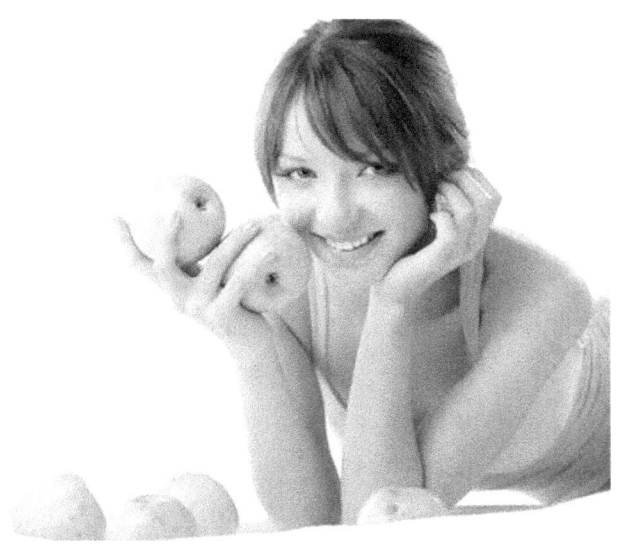

The fact that you're eating clean doesn't mean you should avoid chocolate completely. Everybody loves to have a taste of some fine dessert, at least once in a while. Here are some propositions for sweet desserts you can use when living clean eating lifestyle.

**Chocolate Whoopie Pies**

Ingredients for 32 cookies: dark cocoa powder (5/8 cup, unsweetened), oat flour (1/2 cup), coconut flour (1/4 cup), kosher salt (1/8 tablespoon), stevia in the raw (1 cup), baking soda (1/2 teaspoon), baking powder (1/8 teaspoon), applesauce (2/3 cup, unsweetened), vanilla extract (1/2 teaspoon), 1 egg

Ingredients for filling: Greek yogurt (1/4 cup, unsweetened, unflavored), coconut oil (1/4 cup, chilled), stevia in the raw (2/3 cup), vanilla extract (1 teaspoon)

Preheat your oven to 325°F. Put all dry ingredients in a bowl and mix them up with a whisk. Take another bowl and put in all wet ingredients, mixing them with a whisk or a mixer. Carefully, put the dry ingredients mixture into the wet ingredients, while whisking all the time. Once your batter has dough-like consistency, you're done whisking. Line a baking sheet with parchment paper and drop small dough balls onto it with a spoon. Bake for approximately 15-20 minutes.

Make the filling by combining coconut oil and yogurt, using a stand mixer for about 5 minutes to combine them. Then slowly add stevia and vanilla and mix them in with your mixer set to low and put into the refrigerator for 2 hours. Then simply put the filling between two baked cookies and voila, you have your dessert!

**Banana Bread**

Ingredients: whole wheat pastry flour (1 1/2 cup), baking powder (1 1/4 teaspoon), baking soda (1/2 teaspoon), ground cinnamon (1/2 teaspoon), 2 egg whites (slightly beaten), 3 ripe bananas (1 cup, mashed), stevia in the raw (1/2 cup), coconut oil (1/4 cup), sea salt (1/16 teaspoon)

Preheat your oven to 325-350°F. Use olive oil spray to coat a loaf pan and set it aside. Mash bananas in one bowl and take another bowl to mix flour, baking powder, baking soda, cinnamon, and sea salt. When well combined, set aside. Use the third bowl for mixing egg whites, banana, coconut oil, and sucanat. Once the ingredients are well combined, add flour mixture and stir nicely, until the batter is lumpy. Spoon into the pan and let it bake for around 45 minutes.

**Clean Apple Pie**

Ingredients for pie crust: almond flour (2 cups), zest of lemon, sea salt (1/2 teaspoon), coconut oil (2 tablespoons), 1 egg

# CLEAN EATING BASICS

Ingredients for filling: baking apples (crisp, 3 lbs), lemon juice (3 tablespoons), almond flour (3 tablespoons), vanilla extract (1 teaspoon), ground cinnamon (2 teaspoons), vanilla extract (1 teaspoon), ground cloves (half teaspoon), nutmeg (half a teaspoon), allspice (half teaspoon), light butter (diced and chilled, 2 tablespoons), honey (1/2 cup)

Preheat your oven to 325-350°F. Use a food processor for blending almond flour with salt. Then add the other crust ingredients and process until you see dough is formed. Put it in a pan, cover with wet cloth, and set aside. Take a big bowl and fill it with water before adding 2 tablespoons of juice from lemon. Slice and peel all of the apples and put them in water to keep from browning. Once they are soaking, you need to drain water and wipe the apples with a cloth to dry them. Add the rest of the ingredients, including lemon juice that remained, and toss it all. Transfer apple mixture into the pan with dough and bake for around 45 minutes. Cool before serving.

# CHAPTER FIFTEEN-

# CLEAN EATING MAIN COURSE (ENTREE) RECIPES

Some people think it is hard to eat healthy, because you can't enjoy a truly tasty dish. This is absolutely not true, as there are numerous meals you can prepare that will be delicious and good for your organism. Check out some suggestions.

**Plantain Chips Turkey and Veggie Meatballs**

Ingredients: plantain chips (4 oz), 1/2 of a yellow onion, fresh garlic (2 cloves), fresh ginger (one-inch piece, peeled), celery (4 stalks with trimmed ends), carrots (2 large, trimmed ends, peeled), 1/2 of a zucchini, fresh parsley (1/4 cup), ground turkey (1 pound, organic), coconut aminos (1 teaspoon), fish sauce (1 1/2 teaspoon), sea salt (1 teaspoon), ground sage (1 teaspoon)

## CLEAN EATING BASICS

Preheat your oven to 400°F. Use parchment paper or foil to line a baking sheet. Use a food processor to process plantain chips and set them aside. Put onion, ginger, and garlic in the food processor and blend until nicely chopped, before transferring them to a large bowl.

The next mixture that goes into the food processor is celery, zucchini, carrots, and parsley. When nicely blended, combine with the ginger/garlic/onion mixture. Add ground turkey, fish sauce, coconut aminos, ground sage, and sea salt. Mix them nicely until they are well-combined. Slowly fold in plantain chips you crushed with the new mixture (you can use a spoon). Form meatballs with 1/4 cup measuring cup and place them on the baking sheet. Bake for around 20 minutes, flip and bake for additional 15 minutes until they reach golden brown color.

### Black Bean Plantain Veggie Burgers With Avocado

Ingredients: 1 plantain (ripe), virgin coconut oil (1 teaspoon), black beans (1 can, drained, rinsed), hemp seeds (1/4 cup), tahini (1 1/2 tablespoon), fresh lime juice (1 tablespoon), red onion (1/4 cup, chopped), cilantro (2 tablespoons, chopped), oat flour (1 tablespoon), kosher salt (1/4 teaspoon), chipotle powder

(1/4 teaspoon), virgin coconut oil (1 teaspoon), spouted grain buns

Slice plantains to thin rounds. Add coconut oil to a skillet and warm it over high heat. Add the rounds of plantain and cook each side for maximum 2 minutes, until they get a bit brown. Remove plantains and take 1 cup of the rounds and put it into a large bowl. Add black beans, salt, tahini, chipotle powder, onion, cilantro, lime, and oat flour. Mash it nicely, until all the beans are mashed and split. Warm your skillet over medium heat and add 1 teaspoon of oil. Turn up to high heat, take patty mixture, and form round patties, which you will put in the hot skillet. Each side should be cooked until it browns, for no more than 2 or 3 minutes. Move on until you used all of the mixture. Transfer the patties to the oven, set to 350°F, and bake for additional ten minutes.

You can use vegan mayo, sliced onion, avocado or lettuce, and salsa as a topping. The suggestion is to split a bun in half, put the patty and toppings you want in the middle and serve.

www.ingramcontent.com/pod-product-compliance
Lightning Source LLC
Chambersburg PA
CBHW071117280526
45787CB00003B/1080